SKINCARE TREATMENTS

Proven Solutions For All Skin Types, Glowing Skin DIY For Every Phase Of Life

How To Address Acne, Aging, Sensitivity, Effective Treatments And Essential Tips For Radiant Skin

MAVERICK JENKINS

TABLE OF CONTENTS

INTRODUCTION

A Journey to Healthier Skin

In our search for clear, healthy skin, we can become lost in a sea of products and trends, each claiming to be the next great thing. But skincare is about more than simply goods; it's a personal journey that takes comprehension, patience, and perseverance. This book will help you understand the "why" behind each step, allowing you to design routines that truly work for you.

Our skin is the greatest organ in our bodies, and it is continually influenced by our surroundings, lifestyle, and general health. It represents both our physical and emotional states. When we choose to care for our skin carefully, we are investing in our health, confidence, and comfort in our own skin. This book is intended to equip you with that knowledge and revolutionize the way you look and care for your skin.

Understanding Skin Health

Skin health is fundamentally about maintaining equilibrium. Each layer of skin has an important purpose, ranging from environmental protection to moisture and temperature regulation. The skin's surface is covered in a distinct microbiome of bacteria and other organisms that help defend against hazardous diseases and maintain our skin operating properly.

Skin's Protective Barrier

How the skin barrier keeps moisture in and dangerous substances out, and why maintaining this balance is critical.

The Microbiome's Role

A look at the skin's "ecosystem" and how it contributes to healthy skin.

- **Cell Regeneration:** How the skin constantly renews itself, and how this process varies over time, particularly with age and lifestyle.

Why Skincare Matters

Skincare is more than just looking beautiful; it's about safeguarding your body's first line of defense. Our skin is exposed to daily stressors such as UV radiation, pollution, temperature changes, and more, which can impair its resilience over time. Proper skincare strengthens this protective barrier, slows the symptoms of aging, and even improves our mental health by instilling confidence in how we show ourselves.

Confidence And Self-Care

The psychological benefits of skincare, as well as the increased self-esteem that comes with clear, healthy skin.

Environmental Protection

How a good regimen can protect your skin from pollution, sun exposure, and other elements that cause aging.

Prevention Over Treatment

The importance of proactive skin care in avoiding expensive and complex treatments later on.

Chapter 1

ANATOMY OF THE SKIN

Understanding your skin's structure is the first step towards creating effective skincare. The skin is made up of three primary layers, each having a distinct function in protecting, sustaining, and regenerating our body's outermost barrier:

The Epidermis
The epidermis is the outermost layer that protects the skin from environmental harm and infections. It's where new skin cells develop and push to the surface, forming a protective layer. This layer also includes melanocytes which generates melanin, a pigment that affects skin tone and offers some UV protection.

The Dermis
The dermis, a thicker layer underneath the epidermis, provides strength and suppleness

to the skin. The dermis includes collagen and elastin fibers,which maintains the skin's structure and rigidity. It also contains blood vessels, sweat glands, and hair follicles , which help to regulate temperature, excrete toxins, and promote hair development.

The Subcutaneous Layer (hypodermis)
The deepest layer, subcutaneous tissue, is mostly made up of fat and connective tissue. It functions as an insulator, conserving body heat and cushioning the muscles and bones. The hypodermis stores energy and protects the skin's deeper layers from harm.

Each of these layers works together to build our skin, which is a sophisticated, tough protection. Proper skincare keeps these layers healthy, enhancing their inherent protective and healing properties.

Skin Microbiome And Immunity
Our skin contains a variety of helpful bacteria, fungi, and viruses known as the skin microbiome. This distinct ecosystem

acts as the skin's first line of defense against dangerous microorganisms, inflammation, and infections.

Protective Function
The microbiome creates a protective barrier on the skin's surface, keeping dangerous organisms from entering and causing illnesses.

immunological Support
A healthy microbiome regulates the skin's immunological response, lowering inflammation and increasing overall resilience.

Environmental Interactions
Pollution, food, and even skincare products may disrupt the microbiome equilibrium. When this balance is broken, problems like dryness, irritation, and breakouts may develop. Maintaining a healthy microbiota with mild cleansers while avoiding harsh chemicals and medicines may boost skin immunity.

Our microbiome's health is vital for clean,
healthy skin, so choosing products that
nourish rather than deplete this delicate
ecology is essential for any skin care
program.

How Aging And Environmental Factors Influence Skin Health

As we get older, our skin gradually changes in texture, suppleness, and moisture retention. Environmental variables including pollution, sunshine, and lifestyle choices hasten these changes, which is why knowing the science of aging skin may aid in its management.

Natural Aging

Cell Renewal

As we age, our body's natural cell turnover rate declines, resulting in a buildup of dead cells on the skin's surface. This may produce dullness and uneven texture.

Collagen And Elastin Loss

A decrease in collagen and elastin synthesis causes the skin to droop and wrinkle over time.

- **Hydration Levels**: Aging skin generates less hyaluronic acid, which

causes dryness and a loss of young
suppleness.

Sun Exposure

UV rays damage collagen and elastin fibers,
causing wrinkles, pigmentation, and skin
cancer. Sun protection is vital for reducing
this harm.

Pollution

Free radicals from pollution may
compromise the skin's barrier, causing
irritation, premature aging, and
pigmentation. Antioxidants in skincare may
assist to neutralize free radicals.

Lifestyle Factors

Smoking, bad eating habits, and a lack of
sleep all contribute to skin aging by limiting
blood flow, depleting key nutrients, and
interfering with healing processes.

A well-rounded skincare program that
includes UV protection, antioxidants, and

hydration may help reduce these effects and maintain skin health long into old age.

Explanation Of Common Skin Concerns: Acne, Aging, Sensitivity, And More

Acne

Acne is one of the most common skin conditions, affecting individuals of all ages. It occurs when the pores get blocked with excess oil, dead skin cells, and germs. Acne may vary from little whiteheads and blackheads to severe cystic acne, which can cause scars. Treatments often include controlling oil production, keeping appropriate skin hygiene, and utilizing substances such as salicylic acid, benzoyl peroxide, and retinoids to unclog pores and decrease inflammation.

Aging

As previously noted, aging skin develops wrinkles, fine lines, and sagging as collagen and elastin levels decline. Common therapies include retinoids,peptides, and antioxidants, which increase collagen formation, enhance elasticity, and protect against future damage. To avoid sun-induced aging, SPF should be used on a regular basis as part of any anti-aging regimen.

Sensitivity

Sensitive skin responds quickly to environmental influences, skincare products, and even dietary changes. Symptoms often include redness, itching, and dryness. Minimalistic regimens with fragrance-free, hypoallergenic products containing soothing substances such as aloe vera, chamomile, and niacinamide are beneficial for sensitive skin. Avoiding strong exfoliants and synthetic perfumes may also help to alleviate discomfort.

Hyperpigmentation

Hyperpigmentation, often known as dark spots, arises when certain regions of the skin develop an excess of melanin as a result of sun exposure, acne scarring, or hormonal changes. Ingredients such as vitamin C, niacinamide, and alpha arbutin help lighten dark spots while sunscreen prevents new ones from appearing.

Drying And Dehydration

Dry skin lacks oils, and dehydrated skin loses fluids. Both may cause tightness, flakiness, and sensitivity. Hydrating serums containing hyaluronic acid, ceramides, and rich moisturizers aid in moisture restoration, while avoiding hot water and harsh cleansers helps to keep skin hydrated.

Eczema & Rosacea

Eczema and rosacea are chronic skin disorders characterized by inflammation, redness, and pain. While both need medical treatment, calming products including colloidal oatmeal, azelaic acid, and calendula may help reduce some symptoms. Maintaining a healthy skin microbiota might also help manage flare-ups.

Chapter 2

IDENTIFYING YOUR SKIN TYPE AND ITS UNIQUE REQUIREMENTS

Understanding your skin type is vital for developing a skincare program that is effective for you. While skin types may change owing to variables such as age, environment, and hormones, they are often classified into five categories: normal, dry, oily, combination, and sensitive.

Normal Skin

Normal skin is balanced, not overly oily or dry, and has few blemishes. Pores are typically tiny and even, and this skin type may accept a wide range of products with little discomfort.

Dry Skin

Dry skin often feels tight and scratchy, particularly after cleaning. It may be flaky, itchy, or sensitive. This type has smaller pores and less natural oil production, thus it's vital to use hydrating and moisturizing products.

Oily Skin

Oily skin is distinguished by an abundance of sebum, particularly in the T-zone (forehead, nose, and chin). It often seems glossy and may be prone to blackheads, whiteheads, and enlarged pores. Oily skin benefits the most from gentle cleaning and oil-regulating products.

Combination Skin

Combination skin occurs when certain areas of your face are dry or normal while others (such as the T-zone) are oily. This type may need a balanced approach, with moisturizing solutions on the drier portions and oil-control treatments on the oilier sections.

Sensitive Skin

Sensitive skin responds quickly to new products, environmental changes, and even particular substances, frequently causing redness, itching, or burning sensations. This skin type responds best to products that are gentle, fragrance-free, and hypoallergenic.

Determining your skin type is the first step toward successful skincare, enabling you to choose products that complement rather than upset your skin's natural equilibrium.

UNDERSTANDING SKIN CONDITIONS AND SKIN TYPES

To prevent incompatible products or routines, distinguish skin types(permanent traits) from skin conditions(temporary or curable difficulties). For example, acne, dehydration, pigmentation, and sensitivity are problems that may affect any skin type, but they do not define the skin itself.

Skin Types

These are usually permanent traits, such as oiliness or dryness, and need regular treatment measures.

Skin Conditions

These are impacted by lifestyle, environment, and stress. Acne, redness, and pigmentation are common conditions that need specific treatment and may change over time.

Understanding whether a worry is a type or a condition allows you to tailor your

skincare regimen more efficiently,
employing basic items for your skin type
and treating particular concerns as required.

Skin Type Quiz And Self-Assessment

1. How does your skin feel a few hours after cleansing?
- A) Comfortable, not tight or oily
- B) Tight and maybe flaky
- C) Shiny, particularly around the T-zone
- D) Mostly comfortable, with some greasy spots in the T-zone.
- E) Irritated or Red

2. Do you see any noticeable pores?
- A)Barely noticeable
- B)Small and fine
- C)Enlarged, particularly in the T-zone
- D)Enlarged in some regions but smaller in others
- E)Red or irritated skin surrounding pores

3. How frequently do you get breakouts?
- A) Rarely
- B) Occasionally, owing to dryness
- C) Frequently, particularly in oily areas
- D) Occasionally, in both dry and oily areas
- E) Frequently, in response to new products or stress.

4. What texture does your skin have?
- A) Smooth and even
- B) Rough or flaky
- C) Oily and shiny
- D) Combination of smooth and oily in certain areas
- E) Red, sensitive or reactive

Based on the answers you provided
Mostly A: Your skin is Normal.
Mostly B: Your skin is dry.
Mostly C: Your skin is oily.
Mostly D: you have Combination Skin.
Mostly E: Your skin is sensitive.

Understanding your skin type empowers you to make more educated skincare decisions.

What Is Best For Each Skin Type

Now that you've identified your skin type, let's look at specialized care plans designed to fit your specific requirements.

Normal Skin
- **Routine**:Gentle cleansers, light moisturizers, and daily sunscreen enough to preserve balance.

To keep your skin looking bright, exfoliate once a week and apply antioxidant serums to protect it from environmental assaults.

Dry Skin

For dry skin, use moisturizing cleansers and rich creams with hyaluronic acid, glycerin, and ceramides.

Avoid hot water, which may remove natural oils, and use a moisturizing mask once a week to increase moisture levels.

Oily Skin
- Routine: Use gel-based cleansers, lightweight, oil-free moisturizers, and

products containing salicylic acid to manage oil.
Use clay masks to absorb excess oil, and exfoliate with moderate acids on a regular basis to maintain pores clean.

Combination Skin

- Routine: Use a gentle cleanser and tailored treatments, including lightweight moisturizers for the T-zone and heavier creams for dry regions.

Multi-masking (using several masks for different regions) is an efficient way to satisfy the diverse demands of mixed skin.

Sensitive Skin

- Routine:Use fragrance-free, hypoallergenic products with soothing components such as aloe, niacinamide, and chamomile.

To avoid irritation, avoid aggressive exfoliants and always try new products on a patch.

Chapter 3

BUILDING YOUR PERFECT SKINCARE ROUTINE

Creating a skincare routine that works effectively with your skin's unique needs can make all the difference between achieving balanced, radiant skin or struggling with persistent concerns.

Morning vs. Evening Routines: Key Differences

Your skin's needs differ between day and night, making a dual approach to skincare essential for optimal results. A morning routine prepares and protects your skin for the day's challenges, such as UV exposure and pollutants, while an evening routine is about repair and replenishment.

Morning Routine

Cleanse, moisturize, protect. A gentle cleanse removes overnight buildup, while a lightweight moisturizer and SPF provide hydration and protection against environmental stressors. Antioxidants, like Vitamin C serums, can be added to defend against free radicals.

Evening Routine
Cleanse, treat, and deeply nourish. This is the time for heavier treatments and serums that address specific concerns, such as anti-aging or acne. Ingredients like retinoids, peptides, and hydration boosters are most effective in the evening when skin is at rest and in repair mode.

The Basics of A Healthy Routine: Cleanse, Tone, Moisturize, Protect

Every skincare routine should start with these core steps. Each plays a specific role in maintaining healthy skin, providing a balanced foundation that can be customized with targeted products.

Cleanser

A gentle cleanser removes impurities and excess oil without stripping your skin. Depending on your skin type, you may prefer foaming cleansers for oily skin or cream-based cleansers for dry skin.

Toner

A toner helps to balance the skin's pH, tighten pores, and remove any residual impurities. It also preps the skin to better absorb subsequent products. Look for alcohol-free formulas with soothing or hydrating ingredients like rose water, aloe, or witch hazel.

Moisturizer

A good moisturizer locks in hydration and provides a protective barrier. Choose light, oil-free formulas for oily skin and richer, cream-based options for dry skin.

SPF

Sun protection is a non-negotiable step in your morning routine. Broad-spectrum SPF 30 or higher shields your skin from harmful UV rays, preventing premature aging and reducing the risk of skin damage.

The Essentials: Cleanser, Toner, Moisturizer, SPF, And Beauty Tools

From cleansers to SPF, these products form the core of a balanced skincare routine. Adding beauty tools like jade rollers and facial brushes can enhance product absorption and provide a calming experience.

Jade Rollers

Boost circulation, reduce puffiness, and help serums absorb.

Facial Brushes

Exfoliate gently and stimulate blood flow, ideal for a weekly boost.

When To Use Serums, Masks, And Exfoliants

Targeted treatments address specific concerns and can elevate a basic skincare routine. Knowing when and how to incorporate these treatments ensures your skin receives the right care without being overloaded.

Serums

These are concentrated treatments packed with active ingredients like Vitamin C, hyaluronic acid, and peptides. They target issues such as pigmentation, hydration, and fine lines. Use serums after cleansing and toning for maximum absorption.

Masks

Masks deliver a more intensive dose of active ingredients. Clay masks can help detoxify oily skin, while hydrating masks provide moisture for dry skin. Using a mask 1-2 times a week can revitalize the skin.

Exfoliants

Regular exfoliation removes dead skin cells and encourages cell turnover. Choose chemical exfoliants (like AHA or BHA) for a gentle yet effective approach, or use physical scrubs if your skin is resilient.

Limit exfoliation to 2-3 times per week to prevent irritation.

Layering Products: Serums, Oils, And Active Ingredients

Layering skincare products is an art that can maximize their effectiveness. Proper layering allows each product to penetrate effectively and prevents potential irritation. Here's a general guideline:

Order Of Application

Apply products from thinnest to thickest consistency. Start with water-based serums and toners, then move to thicker creams and oils.

Compatible Ingredients

Some ingredients complement each other, like Vitamin C with Vitamin E, while others should be used separately. For example, retinoids and Vitamin C can cause irritation if layered, so it's best to use them at different times (Vitamin C in the morning, retinoids at night).

Timing Matters
Give each product a moment to absorb
before applying the next, especially if it's an
active treatment.

SAMPLE ROUTINES FOR DIFFERENT SKIN TYPES

Normal Skin
- Morning: Cleanser, toner, antioxidant serum (optional), moisturizer, SPF
- Evening: Cleanser, serum (hydrating or anti-aging), moisturizer

Dry Skin
- Morning: Hydrating cleanser, toner, moisturizer with hyaluronic acid, SPF
- Evening: Gentle cleanser, hydrating serum, rich moisturizer, overnight mask (1-2 times weekly)

Oily Skin
- Morning: Gel cleanser, toner, lightweight moisturizer, SPF
- Evening: Foaming cleanser, salicylic acid serum, oil-free moisturizer, clay mask (1-2 times weekly)

Combination Skin

- Morning: Mild cleanser, toner,
  lightweight moisturizer on T-zone,
  SPF
- Evening: Cleanser, serum (hydrating
  for dry areas, oil-control for T-zone),
  moisturizer

Sensitive Skin
- Morning: Gentle, fragrance-free
  cleanser, hydrating toner, soothing
  moisturizer, mineral SPF
- Evening: Same gentle cleanser,
  hydrating serum (with ingredients like
  aloe or niacinamide), fragrance-free
  moisturizer

Chapter 4

ACNE SOLUTIONS FOR ALL SKIN TYPES

Acne affects individuals of all ages and skin kinds, but knowing the underlying reasons and the best treatments for your specific skin type is critical to getting cleaner skin.

Causes Of Acne
Hormonal,Nacterial, Dietary, And Environmental Factors
Acne's causes may be complicated and multifaceted. Recognizing these factors might help you choose the most effective treatment option.

Hormonal Factors
Hormones, particularly androgens, may cause excessive oil production, blocking pores and resulting in outbreaks. This is why

acne often appears during puberty, menstrual cycles, or periods of stress.

Bacterial Causes
Propionibacterium acnes, or P. acnes, is a common bacterium linked to acne. When pores get blocked, these bacteria may multiply, causing discomfort and outbreaks.

Dietary Influences
High-glycemic meals, such as sugary snacks and dairy, have been associated to acne in certain people. Some individuals may find that changing their eating habits helps them avoid outbreaks.

Environmental Factors
Pollution, dampness, and exposure to harsh chemicals may worsen acne. Comedogenic skincare products, or those that block pores, may also cause outbreaks.

Treating Acne On Oily Or Dry Skin

Acne care involves various techniques based on your skin type. Here's how to customize your treatment:

Oily Skin

Oil-control compounds, such as salicylic acid, may effectively remove excess oil from pores. Gel-based cleansers and oil-free moisturizers are good, while non-comedogenic products aid to avoid more blockage.

Dry Skin

Gentle acne treatments are recommended to maintain moisture levels. Choose moisturizing acne treatments with hyaluronic acid and mild acne-fighting chemicals.

Key Ingredients That Work (Salicylic Acid, Benzoyl Peroxide, And Retinoids)

These potent chemicals are recognized for their acne-fighting properties. Each operates differently, so knowing them will help you choose the best one for your requirements.

Salicylic Acid
This oil-soluble BHA (beta hydroxy acid) effectively unclogs pores and reduces irritation. It is very useful for oily and acne-prone skin.

Benzoyl Peroxide
Eliminates P. acnes germs from the skin's surface. It works well for moderate to severe acne, but it may be drying, so mix it with a moisturizing moisturizer.

Retinoids
Retinoids, such as retinol or prescription-grade tretinoin, increase skin cell turnover, reduce congested pores, and

prevent breakouts. They're great for
long-term acne treatment and may even
enhance skin texture.

Niacinamide And Tea Tree Oil These
anti-inflammatory compounds help soothe
inflamed skin, decrease redness, and
regulate oil production. Niacinamide is very
effective for sensitive skin, and tea tree oil is
a popular natural cure.

Lifestyle Changes To Prevent Breakouts

Lifestyle decisions have a huge impact on acne control.

Dietary Choices
Reducing sugar and high-glycemic meals may help some persons with acne. Increased consumption of anti-inflammatory foods, such as leafy greens, may result in cleaner skin.

Maintain proper skincare and hygiene. Washing pillows on a regular basis, sanitizing phone screens, and keeping hands away from your face may all help to decrease your exposure to acne-causing germs. A twice-daily cleaning practice is vital for removing pollutants and preventing blockage.

Stress Management
High stress levels may lead to hormonal changes that aggravate acne. Yoga,

meditation, and exercise may help you manage stress (and breakouts).

Hydration And Sleep
Staying hydrated promotes skin health, while adequate sleep balances hormones, which are crucial for managing acne.

DIY AND NATURAL ACNE CONTROL

While over-the-counter medications are useful, natural solutions may also assist with mild to severe acne, particularly when taken on a regular basis.

Honey And Cinnamon Mask
Honey has antimicrobial effects, whilst cinnamon is anti-inflammatory. Together, they may assist to minimize redness and germs on the skin. Mix one tablespoon raw honey with a sprinkle of cinnamon, use as a mask for 10-15 minutes, and then rinse.

Green Tea Toning Mist
Green tea contains antioxidants and anti-inflammatory chemicals that soothe sensitive skin. Brew a cup, let it cool, and then apply it as a toner to reduce redness and balance oil.

Apple Cider Vinegar Toner
This natural astringent may regulate skin pH and minimize oil. Combine one part apple

cider vinegar and three parts water, apply
with a cotton pad, and rinse after a few
minutes.

Aloe Vera
With its soothing characteristics, aloe vera
helps reduce inflammation and redness
associated with acne. Apply pure aloe vera
gel to the afflicted regions, leave for 10
minutes, and then rinse.

Chapter 5

ANTI-AGING ESSENTIALS

Aging is a normal process, yet our skin typically shows the most evident symptoms of our age.

Age And Skin: Causes And Early Signs
Skin aging may be attributed to both intrinsic (natural) and extrinsic (external) causes. Knowing the early warning signs might help you begin therapy before fine lines turn into deeper wrinkles.

Intrinsic Aging refers to natural aging caused by decreased collagen formation and cell regeneration. This results in thinner, drier skin and the progressive appearance of fine wrinkles.

Extrinsic Aging
External causes such as sun exposure, pollution, and lifestyle choices (e.g.

smoking, stress) may accelerate skin aging. Sun damage is a major cause, causing dark patches and rough skin texture.

Early Signs To Watch For
Fine wrinkles around the eyes and lips, dullness, minor sagging, and uneven skin tone are all early warning signs that anti-aging treatments should begin.

Anti-Aging Powerhouses: Retinol, Peptides, Antioxidants, Hyaluronic Acid, And Vitamin C

The correct components may have a transformational effect on aged skin.

Retinol
Retinol, a vitamin A derivative, increases cell turnover and collagen formation. This produces smoother, firmer skin with less apparent wrinkles. Retinol is particularly efficient in reducing the appearance of fine lines and improving skin texture over time.

Peptides

These tiny proteins stimulate collagen and elastin production, which are essential for young skin. Regular usage may increase firmness and minimize sagging, making the skin seem more toned.

Antioxidants

Antioxidants, such as vitamins C and E, reduce oxidative stress generated by free radicals, which accelerates aging. Vitamin C, in particular, brightens skin, evens out tone, and promotes collagen creation.

Hyaluronic Acid

Hyaluronic acid, known for its exceptional moisture retention properties, keeps skin plump and moisturized, reducing the appearance of fine wrinkles and giving it a young shine.

Vitamin C

This powerful antioxidant combats pigmentation and UV damage. It may brighten the skin, level out the tone, and protect against environmental aggressors.

Fine Lines And Wrinkles

Different sorts of lines need distinct techniques. Here's how to deal with both effectively:

Regular use of retinoids, peptides, and moisturizing serums help reduce fine lines, which are the early stages of wrinkles. Exfoliating using moderate acids, such as glycolic acid, may help stimulate cell renewal and enhance skin texture.

Deeper Wrinkles

Treatments for deeper wrinkles should be focused and rigorous. Consider combining retinol and peptides for collagen support, as well as antioxidant-rich products, to help delay the deepening of lines. Some users may benefit from expert treatments, such as microneedling or fractional laser therapy, to get more substantial results.

Managing Sun Damage And Hyperpigmentation

Sun exposure accounts for up to 80% of noticeable skin aging. Here's how to treat sun-induced aging symptoms:

Apply sunscreen with broad-spectrum SPF on a daily basis to prevent skin aging. Even on overcast days, use SPF to avoid UV damage and possible hyperpigmentation.

Brightening Ingredients such as Vitamin C, niacinamide, and kojic acid may reduce dark spots and level out skin tone. They act by decreasing melanin formation, reducing the appearance of pigmentation.

Exfoliant Acids
Alpha-hydroxy acids, including as glycolic and lactic acids, promote cell turnover and aid in the removal of pigmented cells. Regular exfoliation also improves the penetration of other anti-aging treatments, increasing their effectiveness.

Non-invasive anti-aging procedures explained

For individuals wishing to take their anti-aging regimen to the next level, these non-invasive solutions deliver noticeable effects without the need for surgery:

Botox And Fillers

Botox temporarily relaxes wrinkle-causing muscles, while fillers restore volume in cheeks and beneath eyes. Both are often used to smooth wrinkles and restore a youthful look.

Chemical Peels

These scrape the top layers of skin with different acid intensities, exposing a smoother, fresher layer below. Peels may help improve skin texture, minimize pigmentation, and boost brightness.

Microdermabrasion is a mild exfoliation procedure that eliminates dead skin cells, stimulates circulation, and improves skin texture. It's perfect for people looking for a non-chemical exfoliating option.

Laser Resurfacing

This procedure employs laser energy to promote collagen and remove damaged skin. It is efficient for reducing wrinkles, scars, and pigmentation, but needs considerable downtime.

Tips For Smoother, Youthful, And Radiant Skin At Any Age

A regular skincare regimen, healthy habits, and preventative steps may help you keep glowing skin at any age.

Drinking water and using hydrating products maintains the skin's moisture barrier, vital for plump, young skin.

Skin restores itself while asleep. Make sure you're receiving enough rest to promote collagen formation and cell regeneration.

Balanced Diet And Antioxidants
Including fruits, vegetables, and omega-3 fatty acids in your diet promotes skin health

from inside. Antioxidants, in particular, serve to counteract oxidative damage.

Exercise boosts circulation, bringing oxygen and nutrients to your skin. It also helps to relieve stress, which may slow the aging process.

Consistent SPF Use
Daily sunscreen use protects skin from UV damage and helps prevent premature aging.

Conduct a monthly skin self-assessment. Regularly check your skin for changes in texture, tone, or new pigmentation. This proactive approach allows you to identify concerns early on and alter your routine as required.

Chapter 6

ADDRESSING SENSITIVE AND REACTIVE SKIN

Sensitive skin might seem like an ongoing battle. Whether it's redness, irritation, or sensitivities to common products, maintaining sensitive skin requires careful attention to ingredients, routines, and even lifestyle choices.

Reasons For Skin Sensitivity And Reactivity

A variety of internal and environmental variables may contribute to sensitivity. Identifying these factors is the first step in controlling and soothing reactive skin.

Genetic Predisposition

Sensitive skin is typically inherited, leading to redness, dryness, and irritation.

Weak Skin Barrier

Impaired skin barrier causes irritants to enter readily, causing irritation and sensitivity. Sensitive skin requires a stronger barrier.

Environmental And Lifestyle Factors

Pollutants, severe temperatures, harsh weather, and stress may all increase skin sensitivity. Changes in humidity or prolonged exposure to the sun without protection may also increase skin responsiveness.

Skincare Product Responses

Fragrances, colors, and harsh preservatives in skincare products might cause responses. Selecting the right products is essential for controlling sensitive skin.

Choosing Gentle Ingredients Niacinamide, Aloe Vera, And Ceramides

Sensitive skin requires substances that are soft and calming. Here are some top picks and how they help to keep your skin calm and balanced:

Niacinamide (Vitamin B3)

Niacinamide is recognized for its relaxing effects and is well tolerated by sensitive skin. It helps to minimize redness, enhances the skin barrier, and increases moisture.

Aloe Vera

Aloe vera is a natural calming ingredient that reduces inflammation and gives cooling comfort to inflamed skin. It's perfect for soothing flare-ups and moisturizing dry spots.

Ceramides

Ceramides are lipids that strengthen the skin barrier, particularly for sensitive skin. They prevent moisture loss and protect the skin from external irritants, making it robust and healthy.

Colloidal Oatmeal

This component is often utilized in sensitive skincare due to its calming effects. It may help reduce itching, redness, and other mild irritations that are often linked with eczema.

HOW TO CHOOSE GENTLE PRODUCTS

Choosing the appropriate products may drastically minimize inflammation while keeping your skin relaxed.

Free Of Fragrance And Alcohol
Fragrances and alcohol are typical allergens, particularly in cleansers and toners. Look for goods branded "fragrance-free" and avoid ones with high alcohol content.

Hypoallergenic Formulations
These products are designed to reduce the risk of responses. To limit the risk of irritation, choose products that cater to delicate skin.

Minimal Ingredient Lists
Using fewer ingredients reduces the danger of provoking sensitivity. Avoid too complicated formulae and instead choose products with clear, plain ingredient lists.

Patch Testing New Products

Test new products on a tiny region of skin, such as the inner arm, to discover possible responses before applying to the face.

Tips To Manage Redness And Irritation

Sensitive skin is prone to persistent redness and irritation.

Use Cold Compresses

Applying a cold, moist cloth to inflamed skin helps decrease inflammation and offer immediate relief from flare-ups.

Use anti-inflammatory ingredients, such as green tea extract and chamomile, to reduce redness over time. These are often found in serums, toners, and relaxing masks.

Limit Exfoliation

Excessive exfoliation might worsen sensitive skin. Use light exfoliants just once a week, or choose for products with low

concentrations of moderate acids such as
lactic acid.

Choose a humidifier for dry environments.
Dry air, particularly in the winter, may
exacerbate skin sensitivity. Using a
humidifier at home keeps the air moist,
which is beneficial for sensitive skin.

Effective Treatments For Eczema, Rosacea, And Dermatitis

Specific skin disorders such as eczema, rosacea, and dermatitis need tailored treatment to control symptoms and avoid deterioration.

Eczema

For eczema-prone skin, use thick moisturizers and emollients that seal in moisture. Ingredients such as shea butter and glycerin provide a protective barrier, reducing itching and dryness.

Rosacea

Rosacea demands mild, relaxing remedies without alcohol or harsh chemicals. Niacinamide, azelaic acid, and licorice extract may reduce redness without creating further discomfort.

Dermatitis

Soothing emollients and barrier repair creams are often used to treat this condition. Ceramide-rich ointments and colloidal oatmeal are great for easing symptoms and restoring the skin's natural defenses.

Adjusting Your Routine During Flare-Ups

Flare-ups are unavoidable for sensitive skin, but changing your routine might help you handle them better.

Simplify your routine. During a flare-up, it's better to stick to the essentials. Use a mild cleanser, moisturizer, and SPF while avoiding actives and exfoliants until your skin settles down.

Avoid hot water and steam, as these might increase redness and sensitivity. Use lukewarm water to cleanse, and avoid saunas and hot showers during the reactive period.

Use anti-inflammatory masks. Use a relaxing mask once or twice each week. Look for substances like aloe, chamomile, or centella asiatica, which are recognized for their soothing properties.

Moisturize often to keep skin moisturized during flare-ups. Reapply a soothing moisturizer throughout the day, particularly if your skin is dry or itching.

Limit Sun Exposure: Sensitive skin may react significantly to the sun. If you must go outdoors, put on a physical sunscreen (ideally mineral-based with zinc oxide or titanium dioxide) and protective clothes.

Chapter 7

HYDRATION AND MOISTURIZATION FOR EVERY SKIN TYPE

Hydration and moisturization are essential for keeping healthy, young skin. While these two procedures are sometimes used interchangeably, they play distinct functions in skincare, with each being vital for producing a healthy, balanced complexion.

The Difference Between Hydration And Moisturization

Hydration refers to the water content of skin cells. When cells are hydrated, they enlarge and plump up, resulting in smooth, velvety skin. Even if your skin is naturally oily, dehydrated skin looks drab and has more wrinkles.

Moisturization seals moisture into the skin. Moisturizers include oils and lipids that form a barrier on the skin's surface to prevent water loss and maintain hydration levels. Without enough moisturization, skin may become dry and flaky.

Understanding these ideas allows you to choose the appropriate solutions to address individual requirements, whether your skin is naturally dry, oily, or somewhere in between.

Best Hydrating Ingredients: Hyaluronic Acid, Glycerin, And Panthenol

Hydrating elements attract and hold water in the skin, making it soft and plump.

Hyaluronic Acid
Hyaluronic acid, a skincare powerhouse, can hold up to 1,000 times its weight in water. It is excellent for all skin types, attracting

moisture to the skin and providing an instant plumping effect.

Glycerin

Glycerin is a humectant that draws moisture from the environment into the skin, making it an efficient hydrator while also supporting a strong skin barrier. It is often found in cleansers and moisturizers.

Panthenol (Provitamin B5) Panthenol is known for its soothing and moisturizing effects, which assist to maintain moisture in the skin while enhancing suppleness and elasticity, making it perfect for sensitive and dry skin.

Chosing The Best Moisturizer For Your Skin Type

The ideal moisturizer differs according on your skin type.

For oily or acne-prone skin, choose for lightweight, oil-free moisturizers to avoid clogging pores. Gel-based moisturizers with hyaluronic acid or glycerin are perfect for providing moisture without leaving a greasy residue.

For dry skin, use a heavier cream-based moisturizer with emollients such shea butter, squalane, or ceramides. These substances assist to repair the lipid barrier and prevent moisture loss.

Mixture Skin
For mixture skin, a balanced approach is ideal. Use a lightweight moisturizer containing moisturizing elements, and if required, add a heavier cream to dry regions such as the cheeks.

For sensitive skin, use fragrance-free, hypoallergenic moisturizers with soothing components like aloe vera and ceramides. Avoid using hefty formulas that might irritate delicate skin.

Hydration Tips For Dehydrated And Dull Skin

Even if your skin does not feel dry, it may be dehydrated, giving the impression of tiredness and dullness. Here are some ways for restoring hydration:

Applying serums to slightly wet skin helps hyaluronic acid seal in moisture more efficiently.

Mist Throughout the Day A moisturizing facial mist may revitalize your skin midday, providing a fast burst of hydration and keeping it looking fresh.

Avoid Over-Exfoliation

Over-exfoliation may remove natural oils and aggravate dehydration. Limit your exfoliation to 2-3 times per week and follow with a moisturizing serum or moisturizer.

Invest in a humidifier. In dry conditions or throughout the winter, a humidifier in your home may assist maintain moisture levels in your skin by avoiding excessive water loss.

At-Home DIY Masks For Hydration Boost

DIY masks are an excellent approach to increase your skin's moisture using natural substances.

Aloe And Honey Mask
Combine equal parts aloe vera gel and honey to create a profoundly moisturizing and relaxing mask. Wait 15-20 minutes before rinsing.

Cucumber And Yogurt Mask Combine half a cucumber and a spoonful of yogurt to create a cooling, hydrating mask that minimizes puffiness and enhances moisture.

Avocado And Olive Oil Mask
Mash half an avocado with 1 teaspoon olive oil. This thick, hydrating mask is ideal for dry skin that needs to be hydrated and softened.

Foods That May Cause Skin Issues

Diet may have a big influence on skin health since some foods can cause inflammation, excessive oil production, and breakouts. Here are a few meals to be cautious about:

Sugar

Consuming high-sugar diets may induce insulin surges, resulting in inflammation and acne. Reducing sugar consumption may help reduce breakouts.

Dairy Products

Some people may have exacerbated acne owing to hormones in milk products affecting the skin. Reduced dairy consumption may enhance skin clarity.

Processed meals include chemicals and preservatives that may cause irritation and damage skin tone and texture over time.

Alcohol

Dehydration may compromise skin barrier function, causing redness and dryness, especially for sensitive skin types.

Example Skin–Healthy Meal Plan And Recipes

Eating nutrient-dense meals may significantly enhance the look of your skin.

Breakfast: Berry-Nut Oatmeal
Oats, high in fiber, along with antioxidant-rich berries and omega-3-rich almonds, make for an excellent start to the day.

Lunch is Quinoa Salad with Avocado and Spinach. Quinoa is abundant in protein and fiber, while avocado has healthy fats that help keep skin hydrated. Spinach contains vitamins A and C, which promote skin healing and rejuvenation.

Snack: Carrots With Hummus
Carrots are abundant in beta-carotene, which the body turns into vitamin A, promoting healthy skin turnover.

Dinner: Grilled Salmon with Steamed veggies

Salmon contains omega-3 fatty acids that promote skin suppleness, while veggies give antioxidants to prevent free radical damage.

Hydration Boost
Lemon and Mint Water infuse water with lemon and mint to enhance hydration and provide vitamin C for collagen formation.

Chapter 8

STRENGTHENING SKIN IMMUNITY AND RESILIENCE

A robust, resilient skin barrier is essential for protecting your skin from environmental irritants, pollutants, and age-related issues. The skin, like our bodies, has its own immune system that works to preserve health, suppleness, and vibrancy.

Understanding Skin Immunity

Skin immunity is a complicated mechanism that defends against dangerous infections, germs, and environmental stresses. The outermost layer, known as the stratum corneum, serves as a defensive barrier, preventing irritants and pollutants from penetrating deeper into the skin.

The Role Of Langerhans Cells

Langerhans cells are specialized immune cells in the skin that identify and react to dangers, prompting the body to respond to inflammation or damage.

External Stressors And Skin Immunity
Pollution, UV radiation, and harsh products may all deplete this immunity over time, resulting in inflammation, dullness, and premature aging. Building a good skin barrier is critical for mitigating these consequences.

Fortifying The Skin Barrier
- Use moderate, pH-balanced cleansers to avoid stripping the skin's natural oils. Over-cleansing may weaken the barrier, resulting in sensitivity and dryness.

Use Barrier Repairing Ingredients
- Ceramides, fatty acids, and cholesterol are vital for renewing the skin's lipid matrix, which keeps moisture in and irritants out.

- Moisturize regularly to preserve hydration and keep the barrier intact. Choose a moisturizer with skin-type-specific components such as squalane, shea butter, or hyaluronic acid.

The Benefits Of Probiotics For Skin

Probiotics aren't only good for your stomach; they also help to maintain a healthy skin microbiome, which boosts overall immunity.

Boosts healthy bacteria

Probiotics help maintain a healthy microbiome on the skin's surface, eliminating unwanted germs and fostering a better environment. This may help treat acne and eczema by lowering inflammation and redness.

Probiotic skincare may enhance skin texture, making it smoother and more resistant to environmental harm.

Strengthens the skin barrier
Probiotics serve to strengthen the skin's
natural defenses, preventing dangerous
germs from growing and disrupting the skin
barrier.

How To Restore And Maintain A Healthy Skin Barrier

Limit Exfoliation

Excessive exfoliation may decrease the skin barrier, leading to irritation and dryness. Exfoliate 1-3 times a week with mild products, especially if you have sensitive skin.

Incorporate Antioxidants

Vitamin C, green tea extract, and niacinamide help combat free radicals, decrease inflammation, and promote skin regeneration, resulting in a stronger and healthier barrier.

Hydrate With Humectants Ingredients like glycerin and aloe vera attract water to the skin, keeping it hydrated. Proper hydration is critical for maintaining barrier health and minimizing water loss.

Natural Ingredients For Immunity Boost (e.g., Aloe Vera And Green Tea)

Aloe Vera

Aloe vera, known for its soothing and anti-inflammatory characteristics, reduces irritation while also providing moisture, which helps to protect the skin barrier. It is very helpful for delicate or damaged skin.

Green Tea

Green tea contains antioxidants that protect against UV damage and prevent inflammation. Polyphenols aid to repair damaged cells, which improves skin resilience and general health.

Honey

Honey is a natural humectant that maintains moisture and has antibacterial effects to boost skin immunity and prevent breakouts.

Turmeric

Turmeric's anti-inflammatory and antioxidant properties decrease redness and promote healing, making it an ideal option for robust skin.

Centella Asiatica (Cica)

Cica helps to reduce inflammation, promote cell healing, and increase hydration. It is particularly useful for delicate skin types that need barrier protection.

Tips To Maintain Healthy, Resilient Skin

Sun protection is crucial since UV rays may break down collagen and damage the skin barrier. Daily SPF use is required, especially on overcast days, to preserve skin immunity and prevent premature aging.

Stay hydrated from the inside out. Drinking adequate water improves skin health and helps to maintain its natural moisture balance. Hydration promotes all skin processes, including healing and resilience.

Sleep allows the skin to heal itself and renew new cells. Prioritizing regular sleep promotes healthy skin regeneration and strengthens the barrier to everyday pressures.

Avoid overuse of active ingredients. While actives such as retinoids and exfoliants offer advantages, excessive usage might erode the barrier. To prevent undermining the skin's natural defenses, use them in conjunction with calming and moisturizing products.

Adopt a Balanced Diet. Foods high in vitamins, antioxidants, and healthy fats promote skin resiliency. Omega-3 fatty acids, found in fish and flaxseeds, are especially good for strengthening the skin's barrier and lowering inflammation.

Chapter 9

SEASONAL SKINCARE

Every season has a distinct set of problems for our skin, ranging from the drying effects of winter cold to the harsh sun exposure in summer. Understanding how your skin's demands vary with the seasons and how to modify your regimen may make a significant difference in keeping a balanced, healthy complexion.

How Changing Seasons Affect Skin

The skin is continually responding to variations in temperature, humidity, and environmental conditions. Seasonal changes may upend its natural equilibrium, necessitating the use of new treatments and regimens to keep it safe and moisturized.

Winter

Dry air and indoor heating deplete moisture, resulting in flaky, tight, and sensitive skin.

Spring

As the weather warms, your skin may generate more oil and need detoxification to remove the dullness of winter.

Summer

Increased sun exposure, heat, and humidity may cause greasy skin, blocked pores, and sunburn.
Fall: Cooler, drier weather arrives, suggesting the need for a richer, more hydrating regimen to prepare for winter.

Setting Your Routine For Winter, Spring, Summer, And Fall

Winter

Use Rich, Hydrating Products*1
Switch to a Creamy Cleanser. In the winter, gel or foamy cleansers may peel the skin; instead, go for a creamy product that nourishes while cleansing.

Choose a heavier moisturizer containing components such as ceramides, squalane, and shea butter to seal in moisture and preserve the skin barrier.

Add A Humidifier
Indoor heating may dry up the air. Using a humidifier may help keep your skin hydrated.

Spring
Refresh and Brighten

- Exfoliate gently. Spring is the best time to shed winter's drab skin. Use a mild exfoliant with AHAs or BHAs once or twice a week.

Switch To Lightweight Moisturizers

As temps increase, use a lighter moisturizer to avoid oiliness and retain moisture.

Focus on Antioxidants: Serums containing vitamin C, green tea, and ferulic acid may

protect skin from pollution and
environmental stresses.

Summer
Protect and Balance
- Prioritize sun protection. Apply a broad-spectrum SPF 30 or higher every day, and reapply as required. Physical sunscreens with zinc oxide provide excellent protection.

- apply a Mattifying Moisturizer: Summer heat and humidity may generate extra shine, so apply a lightweight moisturizer to reduce oil.

- Use a Hydrating Mist
- A facial mist may refresh and moisturize skin without affecting makeup or SPF.

Fall
Repair and Rehydrate
- Repair Summer Damage

Use antioxidants, retinoids, or peptides to address hyperpigmentation, fine lines, and sun damage from summer.

- Move to heavier Textures
  Use a heavier moisturizer with hyaluronic acid to keep skin hydrated when temperatures drop.

- Consider using sleep masks once or twice a week to improve hydration and barrier restoration.

Special considerations for humidity, cold, and sun exposure
Each weather aspect has specific challenges:

High Humidity
Use non-comedogenic, gel-based moisturizers and a mild SPF. In warm, humid regions, avoid using heavy lotions, which may block pores.

Cold Temperatures

Choose oil-based cosmetics that provide a protective barrier on the skin. To prevent moisture loss, ensure that your moisturizer contains occlusives such as lanolin or petroleum.

Sun Exposure
Year-round sun protection is essential. To combat sun-induced oxidative stress, use hats, sunglasses, and UPF-rated clothes, as well as antioxidant-rich products.

Product Recommendations By Season
Here are some important goods to consider for every season:

Winter
Cream cleanser, heavy moisturizer, hydrating serum, and overnight repair masks.

Spring
Exfoliating toner, lightweight moisturizer, and antioxidant serum.

Summer
Gel-based sunscreen, mattifying moisturizer,
and hydrating facial mist.

Fall
Rich moisturizer, peptide or retinoid serum,
and barrier repair cream.

Sun Protection Year-Round: More Than Just SPF
SPF is important, but a more comprehensive
approach to sun protection improves skin
health and longevity:

- Apply SPF as the last step in your
  skincare process and beneath makeup
  for optimum coverage.

- Use Physical Barriers Wearing hats,
  sunglasses, and UPF-rated clothes
  may give additional sun protection,
  especially on lengthy days.

- Incorporate Antioxidants

Vitamin C and E may minimize oxidative stress and UV damage when combined with SPF.

Traveling Skincare Tip: What To Pack For Different Climates

When traveling, your skin is exposed to a variety of environmental conditions, so bring cosmetics that are appropriate for your destination's temperature.

Multi-Tasking Products

Select products with numerous advantages, like as a moisturizer with SPF, to simplify your regimen and conserve space.

Travel-Friendly Hydrating Mist

Air travel may cause skin to dry out rapidly. A hydrating spray may help keep moisture levels stable during and after flights.

Pack For The Climate

For tropical climates, include lightweight, mattifying products with SPF. Bring thicker moisturizers and moisturizing serums to cooler places.

Portable Sunscreen

Use sunscreen sticks or powders for
on-the-go reapplication, particularly for
longer outdoor activities.

Chapter 10

SKINCARE ACCORDING TO AGE AND LIFE STAGE

Our skin's requirements alter with each life stage, driven by hormonal shifts, environmental circumstances, and personal preferences. Recognizing these transitions enables us to tailor skincare regimens to individual needs at all ages, from adolescent breakouts to mature skin care throughout menopause and beyond.

Teen Skin
Navigating skincare throughout adolescence frequently entails dealing with hormonal changes that cause acne, oiliness, and skin sensitivity. Developing a consistent but mild skincare practice may be revolutionary, aiding in the prevention of long-term skin problems.

Cleansing

Use a mild, sulfate-free cleanser to remove dirt, oil, and impurities without stripping the skin.

Managing Acne

Salicylic acid and benzoyl peroxide are efficient acne treatments, but they should be used with calming substances to reduce inflammation.

Sun Protection

Encourage early SPF usage to avoid sun damage and preserve young skin.
To protect skin from being overwhelmed, avoid vigorous cleaning, stick to a schedule, and keep it simple.

Skin Care For Adults

As we get older, our skin frequently encounters additional problems, such as symptoms of premature aging, uneven skin tone, and environmental damage. This stage benefits from a balanced strategy that prioritizes skin health while avoiding premature aging.

Antioxidants

Use serums high in antioxidants such as vitamin C and E to combat free radicals and brighten the skin.

Moisturization

Choose lightweight, moisturizing products to keep skin lush without clogging pores.

Preventive Treatments

Use retinoids or peptides to boost collagen formation and reduce fine wrinkles. Prioritize protection and maintenance, and avoid overusing items that may disturb the skin barrier.

Menopause & Beyond

Menopause causes major hormonal changes that impact skin elasticity, moisture, and thickness. Skin may thin and dry out, making it more susceptible to sagging and wrinkles. During this stage, caring practices that focus hydration, collagen support, and gentle care are vital.

Rich Moisturizers

To fully nourish the skin, choose moisturizers containing moisturizing components such as ceramides, hyaluronic acid, and peptides.

Collagen-Boosting Ingredients

Retinoids, vitamin C, and peptides may help boost collagen and reduce skin thinning.

Sensitivity Awareness

Menopausal skin may become more sensitive, so avoid harsh substances and go for soft formulations.

To battle dryness and sagging, prioritize products that increase hydration and strengthen the skin barrier.

Pregnancy Safe Skincare: What To Use And Avoid

Pregnancy causes hormonal changes that may alter skin, resulting in irritation, acne, and hyperpigmentation. Safety is a primary consideration, since certain skincare components might be harmful during pregnancy.

Ingredients such as retinoids, salicylic acid, and some essential oils may not be suitable to use while pregnant.
Go For Gentle Alternatives Consider using azelaic acid to treat acne and niacinamide to soothe inflammation and balance skin tone.

SUN PROTECTION

Hormonal fluctuations may make skin more sensitive to UV exposure, thus using SPF on a regular basis is essential for preventing hyperpigmentation.

Keep routines simple, stay hydrated, and speak with a healthcare professional about ingredient safety.

Care For Skin During Illness Or Stress
Illness and stress may damage skin, causing dryness, breakouts, and sensitivity. During these times, skin need additional care, including regimens that focus moisture and comfort.

Soothing components
Choose relaxing components like aloe vera, chamomile, and colloidal oatmeal to alleviate sensitivity and irritation.

Hydration Focus
Drink lots of water and use hydrating serums or creams to keep your skin moisturized, since stress and sickness may dry your body and skin.

Gentle Cleansing

Use a moderate, non-foaming cleanser to prevent causing further irritation during times of susceptibility.

Keep routines simple, prioritize hydration and comfort, and respond to your skin's demands.

Post-Procedure Skincare

What to Use Following Peels, Lasers, and Facials

Cosmetic procedures like chemical peels, laser treatments, and facials may improve skin, but they also need special aftercare to encourage healing and optimize results. Proper post-procedure care protects delicate skin, reduces inflammation, and promotes regeneration.

Hydration And Barrier Support

To restore the skin barrier, use rich moisturizers and serums containing ceramides, hyaluronic acid, and peptides. Avoid retinoids, acids, and exfoliants for a few days after treatment to prevent irritation.

Sun Protection

After treatments, skin is more sensitive, so use a broad-spectrum SPF 30 or higher every day and prevent direct sun exposure. Follow your dermatologist's recommendations, use mild and soothing creams, and prioritize hydration and sun protection.

Chapter 11

THE IMPACT OF DIET, HYDRATION,AND LIFESTYLE ON SKIN

Skin health is affected not just by what we apply outwardly, but also by what we eat and how we live.

Foods That Nourish And Protect Your Skin

Our diets play an important part in skin health because some foods are high in antioxidants, vitamins, and minerals, which help the skin's natural defenses and healing systems.

Antioxidant-Rich Foods

Berries, leafy greens, and nuts are abundant in antioxidants, which help fight free radicals and prevent premature aging.

Omega-3 And Healthy Fats

Fatty fish, chia seeds, and walnuts provide omega-3 fatty acids that improve skin suppleness and moisture by reinforcing the lipid barrier.

Consume vitamin-rich foods for radiance, including as citrus fruits, bell peppers, almonds, sunflower seeds, and sweet potatoes and carrots. These foods encourage collagen creation and repair.

The Importance Of Hydration For Skin Elasticity And Glow
Proper hydration is essential for maintaining skin's moisture balance and suppleness. Dehydrated skin usually appears dull, feels tight, and is prone to fine wrinkles and irritation.

The Importance Of Water Intake
Drinking enough of water helps keep cells hydrated, keeping skin plump and decreasing the appearance of fine wrinkles. For optimum hydration, drink 8-10 cups each day.

Hydrating Foods
Water-rich fruits like cucumbers, melons, and oranges promote hydration and provide vitamins and minerals.

Avoiding Dehydrators
Limit coffee and alcohol consumption since they might dry skin and reduce its resistance. If eaten, drink plenty of water to balance it out.

Skin Care Supplements: Collagen, Vitamins, And Antioxidants
While a balanced diet is recommended, some supplements might provide additional skin advantages, especially if certain nutrients are deficient.

Collagen Supplements
Collagen peptides may improve skin suppleness, minimize wrinkles, and increase moisture from inside. Search for high-quality, bioavailable forms.

Vitamins A, C, D, and E. These vitamins are necessary for skin health. Vitamin C, in particular, stimulates collagen formation, while vitamin D promotes cell healing.

Antioxidants And CoQ10
CoQ10, zinc, and selenium are potent antioxidants that reduce oxidative stress and promote young look.

Stress And Skin: Managing The Connection

Stress may have a negative impact on skin, leading to diseases such as acne, eczema, and premature aging. Learning to handle stress has a favorable influence on both mental and skin health.

Stress-related Skin Issues

High cortisol levels caused by stress may result in increased oil production, breakouts, and inflammation. Chronic stress lowers the skin's barrier, leaving it more vulnerable to injury.

Mindful Practices For Better Skin

Meditation, yoga, and deep breathing are all relaxing techniques that may help your skin be more resilient. Consistent sleep is also necessary for skin healing and cell regeneration.

Lifestyle Adjustments

Regular exercise improves circulation and oxygen flow, resulting in a natural glow.

Avoid smoking, since it hastens aging and destroys collagen.

Sample Meal Plans For A Skin-Friendly Diet

A well-balanced diet geared toward skin health may be both pleasant and nutritious. Here are some example meal plans to help you easily include skin-boosting nutrients and water into your daily routine.

Breakfast

Smoothie with berries, spinach, almond milk, chia seeds, and collagen powder. Whole-grain avocado toast with pumpkin seeds and chili flakes.

Lunch

Grilled salmon or tofu salad with mixed greens, bell peppers, and citrus vinaigrette. Lentil soup served with a cucumber and tomato salad.

For a snack, try fresh fruit with nuts or a green drink with kale, celery, and apple.

Dinner

Stir-fried vegetables with quinoa, sweet potatoes, and turmeric.Spiced grilled chicken served with whole wheat pasta, spinach, cherry tomatoes, garlic, olive oil, and nutritional yeast.

Hydration

Enjoy infused water with lemon, cucumber, or mint throughout the day to stay hydrated.

Chapter 12

TARGETED AND ADVANCED THERAPIES

Advanced therapies and tailored treatments are effective solutions for anyone wanting a more rigorous skincare regimen. These treatments may address issues including as aging, scarring, hyperpigmentation, and uneven texture, using both in-office procedures and effective at-home devices.

Advanced skincare treatments have developed to provide extremely tailored outcomes. Here is a summary of some of the most popular treatments available today:

Microneedling (collagen induction treatment) creates regulated micro-injuries in the skin to stimulate collagen and elastin formation. This therapy is helpful in improving skin texture, reducing acne scars, and brightening overall skin tone.

Chemical Peels

A solution is used to thoroughly exfoliate the skin, eliminating dead layers and revealing smoother, fresher skin below. Peels vary from light to deep, addressing pigmentation, sun damage, fine wrinkles, and dullness.

Laser Treatments

Fractional lasers and intense pulsed light (IPL) employ particular light wavelengths to treat skin issues. They may minimize redness, sun spots, acne scars, and symptoms of age, therefore enhancing the overall look of your skin.

Benefits And Risks Of Office Procedures

Each sophisticated treatment offers distinct advantages, but it also has hazards that must be carefully considered. Consultation with a skilled specialist guarantees that you make the best option for your skin.

The Advantages Of In-Office Treatments

- Targeted, customized, and usually more effective than topical therapies.
- Rapid recovery for mild to moderate treatments.
- Long-term outcomes with constant care

Risks To Consider

- Side effects may include redness, irritation, swelling, or hyperpigmentation.
- If not administered by a skilled practitioner, there is a risk of infection or scarring. Recovery time varies depending on therapy.

At-Home Devices: What Works And What Does Not

With developments in skincare technology, numerous at-home gadgets now offer professional-quality results. However, not all are equally effective, and some might be dangerous if overused.

Effective At-Home Devices
LED Light Therapy Devices
These devices employ light at various wavelengths to treat acne, decrease inflammation, and increase collagen production. Blue light reduces acne-causing germs, and red light promotes anti-aging.

Microcurrent Devices
These devices use low-level electrical currents to tone and tighten face muscles, resulting in a tighter look with regular usage.

Equipment To Use With Caution
- Microneedling Rollers:Although some promise advantages for texture, at-home rollers lack the accuracy of professional equipment, raising the risk of infection and discomfort.

- Dermaplaning Tools:Used for exfoliation; however, incorrect technique may result in wounds or discomfort.

Avoid devices such as high-intensity lasers and peels. These are best left to specialists since overuse might result in serious burns or pigmentation disorders.

When To Visit A Dermatologist

Knowing when to see a dermatologist is vital for maintaining good skin health. Professional counsel may help to avoid problems and ensure that treatments are appropriate for your skin type and concerns.

Persistent Skin Concerns
If over-the-counter medicines and at-home cures fail to alleviate acne, eczema, or chronic redness, it may be necessary to see a dermatologist.

Specialized Concerns (e.g., Scarring, Deep Wrinkles)
Dermatologists provide safe and effective treatments for scarring, hyperpigmentation, and indications of aging.

Routine Skin Health Checks
Yearly skin screenings may detect skin cancer and other abnormalities early.

Regular checkups promote proactive and preventative treatment.

Choosing The Best Treatment For Your Concerns

With so many alternatives available, it's critical to customize treatments to your skin type, problems, and lifestyle.

Identify Your Goals

Determine if your main problem is acne, age, pigmentation, or texture. This clarity enables you and your dermatologist to devise a focused strategy.

Consider recovery time, including any necessary break for recovering. Deeper chemical peels and laser treatments, for example, may need a week or more of recovery time.

Budget considerations

Advanced therapies may be pricey. Consider treatments that provide the best value for

your objectives, as well as maintenance
choices that are within your budget.

Chapter 13

DIY REMEDY AND NATURAL SKINCARE

Choosing natural skincare may be both empowering and cost-effective. Creating bespoke solutions at home allows you to manage the ingredients, eliminate chemicals, and adapt each cure to your skin's individual requirements.

Benefits And Risks Of DIY Skincare

Benefits Of DIY Skincare

- Cost-Effective:Homemade skincare solutions are often less costly than commercial goods.

- Ingredient Control:Customize ingredients to meet your skin's specific requirements while avoiding irritants and allergies.

- Eco-Friendly:Minimizes packaging waste, making it a sustainable option.

Risks Of DIY Skincare

- Allergies or Irritation:Some natural products may cause irritation or allergic responses.

- Short Shelf Life:Because DIY goods lack preservatives, they should be used immediately to avoid deterioration and bacterial development.

- Variability Of Results:Results may vary depending on component quality, application consistency, and skin type.

Effective Natural Ingredients And How To Use Them

Natural substances, when applied right, may have strong outcomes. Here are some of the more effective alternatives, along with their benefits:

Aloe Vera

Aloe vera, known for its calming and anti-inflammatory characteristics, helps reduce redness, hydrate the skin, and aid healing. Use it as a basis for masks or a mild moisturizer.

Honey

Honey, a natural humectant, attracts moisture to the skin while also providing antimicrobial effects, making it great for acne-prone skin. Apply straight or combine with other items to create a moisturizing mask.

Oatmeal

Oatmeal is soothing for sensitive skin and relieves inflammation. It may be pounded into powder for use in masks and scrubs.

Tea Tree Oil

Tea tree oil is known for its antimicrobial characteristics and may help with acne problems. To prevent irritation, dilute it with a carrier oil (such as jojoba oil).

Green Tea

Green tea contains antioxidants that help battle free radicals and decrease inflammation. Use brewed, cooled tea as a toner, or include green tea powder into masks.

DIY Face Masks, Toners, And Moisturizers For All Skin Types

Creating personalized goods allows you to address unique skin concerns. The following recipes are suited to each skin type:

For Oily And Acne-Prone Skin

Charcoal and Tea Tree Mask. To make a paste, combine 1 teaspoon activated charcoal, a few drops of tea tree oil, and a little water. Apply, let to rest for 10 minutes, then rinse off.

For Dry Skin

Honey and Avocado Mask. Mash 1/4 avocado and add with 1 tablespoon honey.

Apply for 15-20 minutes, then rinse for more hydration.

For Sensitive Skin
oats and Yogurt Mask: Combine 1 tablespoon ground oats and 2 tablespoons plain yogurt. Apply for 10-15 minutes to reduce discomfort.

For combination skin
Green Tea and Aloe Toner. Brew green tea, chill, then combine with aloe vera gel. Apply a cotton pad for a refreshing toner.

How To Make Natural Products Last

Because DIY goods lack preservatives, understanding how to store them is critical for safety and effectiveness.

Little Batches
Prepare little quantities that may be consumed within a week or two.

Refrigeration
Keep items in the refrigerator, particularly those containing perishable components such as yogurt or fruit.

Sterilize Containers
Thoroughly clean the containers to prevent bacteria accumulation.

Avoid Contamination
To avoid spoiling, apply DIY items using clean hands or utensils.

Safely incorporating essential oils and plant extracts

Essential oils may enhance your DIY skincare, but they need cautious handling.

Always dilute essential oils with a carrier oil, such jojoba or almond oil, to prevent irritation.

Patch Test

Before applying a new oil, put a little quantity to your inner arm and wait 24 hours to verify no response.

Popular Essential Oils

Lavender:Calms and soothes skin, especially sensitive skin.

Rosehip: High in antioxidants; excellent for anti-aging.

Chamomile: Reduces irritation and is good for redness-prone skin.

Sample Recipes For Skincare Essentials

Apply Calming Lavender Face Mist. Mix 1/2 cup pure water, 5 drops lavender essential oil, and 1 teaspoon aloe vera gel.

Pour into a spray bottle to create a pleasant mist.

Brightening Turmeric Mask

Combine 1/2 tsp turmeric powder, 1 tbsp yogurt, and a few drops of honey. Apply for 10 minutes, then rinse completely to enjoy the shine.

Coconut & Sugar Scrub

Combine 1/2 cup coconut oil and 1/2 cup sugar to make a light exfoliating scrub. Apply weekly for soft, smooth skin.

Chapter 14

RESOLVING COMMON SKIN ISSUES

While everyone's skin is different, many of us encounter similar issues that may affect our skin's look and health.

How To Treat Dark Spots And Hyperpigmentation

Sun exposure, hormone fluctuations, and prior acne are all common causes of dark patches and hyperpigmentation. Here's how to minimize their appearance:

Exfoliation For Increased Cell Turnover
Regular exfoliation with AHAs (such as glycolic acid) or BHAs (such as salicylic acid) induces new skin cells to replace discolored ones, resulting in the gradual disappearance of dark spots.

Brightening Ingredients

- Vitamin C: An antioxidant that reduces dark spots and combats free radicals. Use in the morning for the greatest effects.

- Niacinamide: This type of Vitamin B3 helps to diminish pigmentation and level out skin tone lol

- **Licorice Root Extract** Naturally brightens skin and minimizes the appearance of dark spots.

Sun Protection

Use SPF consistently to prevent hyperpigmentation. Apply a broad-spectrum SPF every day to prevent additional discoloration and protect treated areas.

Managing Larger Pores

Excess oil production and plugged pores are two common causes of enlarged pores. To reduce their appearance, keep pores clean and minimize grease.

Use gentle exfoliation with salicylic acid to clear pores and decrease their appearance. Look for BHA-based toners and masks.

Oil Control

Clay masks remove excess oil and purify pores. Use once a week, concentrating on the T-zone and oily regions.

Retinoids

Retinoids increase cell turnover and prevent pores from expanding. If you are new to retinoids, start with a low concentration and just use them at night.

Hydration

Proper hydration balances oil production and reduces pore visibility. Choose lightweight, noncomedogenic moisturizers.

Solutions For Dry And Flaky Skin

Weather changes, dehydration, and using harsh skincare products may all cause dry patches and flaky skin. Here's how to moisturize and smooth dry skin:

Humectant-Rich Products Hyaluronic acid and glycerin bring moisture to the skin. To seal in moisture, layer a moisturizing serum before your moisturizer.

Barrier Repairing Moisturizers Ceramides and fatty acids help rebuild the skin barrier and prevent moisture loss.

Avoid Harsh Cleansers
Choose mild, sulfate-free cleansers that do not deplete the skin's natural oils, which may aggravate dryness.

Weekly Hydrating Masks
Apply a hydrating mask once or twice a week to increase skin moisture levels. Look for components such as aloe vera, honey, and chamomile.

Addressing Dullness And Uneven Texture

Dull skin and rough texture are generally caused by a buildup of dead skin cells, dehydration, or a lack of exfoliation. Restore your skin's shine by following these steps:

Exfoliation For Radiance
Regular exfoliation (chemical or manual) eliminates dead skin cells, resulting in brighter, smoother skin. Glycolic acid is extremely good in reducing dullness.

Vitamin C for Glow
Vitamin C serums brighten and enhance skin texture over time. If you have sensitive skin, choose stable versions such as sodium ascorbyl phosphate.

Hydration
Dehydrated skin may seem dull. To plump and smooth skin, use a hydrating serum first, followed by a moisturizer.

Facial Massage

Using a jade roller or gua sha tool helps
improve circulation, give skin an immediate
glow, and aid in lymphatic drainage.

Practical Tips For Long-Term Results

Consistency and a deliberate approach to skincare may boost your results and keep your skin healthy over time.

Maintain a consistent regimen to avoid skin irritation. Maintain a steady, effective regimen and allow items time to work.

Patch Test New Products
Test new products on a tiny area to prevent discomfort, particularly when addressing specific conditions.

Sleep And Stress Management
Sleep and stress have a big influence on skin health. To maintain the resilience of your skin, prioritize relaxation and stress-reduction exercises.

Hydration Inside And Out

Maintain a nutritious diet with fruits, vegetables, and healthy fats to enhance your skin's natural radiance.

Seek professional treatment for chronic skin disorders. They may prescribe in-office treatments like as chemical peels, microneedling, or laser therapy to improve outcomes.

CONCLUSION

The quest for better skin is much more than simply applying products,it's about recognizing and respecting your specific skin requirements. As you approach the conclusion of your trip through the layers, routines, and solutions of successful skincare, keep that in mind. From hydration and resilience to acne and aging, this book has you covered. You can now make informed decisions and create a regimen that works for you because of the information, resources, and insights it provides.

The process of skincare is just as important as the end result. The idea is to turn skincare into a ritual that boosts your confidence and skin health, rather than a mundane task, by adopting a more meaningful kind of self-care. Your skin, in all its uniqueness, needs care and respect, and this message is reinforced with each chapter, regimen, and little act of maintenance.

As you apply what you've learned, keep in mind that achieving healthy, glowing skin is an ongoing process that is unique to you and always changing. Things like the seasons, your demands, and technological advancements are subject to change. Always pay attention to your skin's signals, maintain your curiosity, and be consistent.

You are now equipped to tackle the ever changing skincare industry with the information and resources provided here. May each step in your path not only lead to better skin but also to a restored feeling of self-assurance and delight in caring for the face you display to the world every day.